Acknowledgements

I want to thank my good friend Marc Paul Kaplan, author of multiple award-winning Chasing Klondike Dreams, for his insights and helpful editing and my friend Jim Greenwood, entrepreneur, for his insights on delivering the promise spelled out in Chapter One. I want to thank Chris Padula for the covers he always creates for me. ctenel@tlen.pl. I wish to thank friends for their helpful ideas and support.

Other books:

The Good Life Plan

Making Every Day Count

The Surfing Life

Table of Contents

Foreword

This book is a Course for review by business executives looking for a more comprehensive approach to creating happy workers. It is a full body, mind, and spirit approach to helping workers find fulfillment, reduce stress, and cultivate mental and physical health.

For workers it is a guideline to incorporating certain behaviors into your daily lives to develop your potential, find purpose, feel life is meaningful, become healthy, and understand happiness.

We are born to be happy. We are born to be healthy. But health and happiness are not always how the advertising media and story books portray it. Health and Happiness are Nature's goal in seducing us to seek behaviors that enhance our survival opportunities. In Nature, we are still early man and all animals are seduced with happiness brain chemicals to engage in activities that ensure survival of their species.

The neurotransmitters and hormones of happiness are stimulated by intentions, actions, successes, and health. We spend our lives chasing ideals we think will create life-long happiness. There is no need to chase ideals for years. Happiness is readily available if you accept what it is. We can experience it every day with the behaviors Nature intended us to pursue.

Workers want to feel purposeful, reduce stress, have work life balance, and increase their promotion opportunities. They can learn to initiate the right behaviors to enhance each of these goals on their own. That is the purpose of this Course. Achieving these goals through the right behaviors is Nature's plan for enhancing survival and her rewards include stimulating happiness.

We will cover these habits and learn to engage in the right positive behaviors that can have immediate results. We can begin today just by having the right intentions and planning to engage in some positive behaviors.

We will unlock the easy to access secrets in every person's DNA. We may think we have to be rich and famous to be happy. We don't.

Even the rich and famous have to continue their growth to maintain their feelings of euphoria. This is why so many people self-destruct after achieving what should be their dream. They imagined one event or achievement would take care of happiness for the rest of their lives.

The true path of happiness is growth. Riches are often the result, but riches are not the achievement that sustains happiness. Happiness can be present every day without riches and even before achieving the destination we have in mind.

Happiness is the journey more than the destination. Happiness is finding the daily habits that promote our survival opportunities and leaving the destination to unfold in due course.

The reward of happiness comes during planning, executing, and enjoying our progress. This process including health and exercise stimulate all our happiness brain chemicals. Once we have hit a summit, we then move into the process of reaching the next summit. Reaching summits becomes our goals.

The five behaviors suggested in this Course assist us in finding daily happiness and achieving our personal and career goals. The behaviors are the secret that unlock the happiness in our DNA.

Chapter One

The Promise

The goal of this course is to find happiness every day that will lead to fulfilling your long-term aspirations. Not only is it possible to have happiness every day, it is practical. Our progress is dependent on finding the sweet spot in our careers and our lives so we can stop wasting time and traveling in the wrong directions.

The sweet spot comes from loving what we do and being good at it. The sweet spot is loving our lives and being good at conducting them. Loving our activities is important because it is hard to be passionate without the love. Engaging in the right behaviors will bring in the passion.

Every passionate person has already discovered the secrets. We can do something we are great at, but if we don't love it, we will probably burn out or find something that is more rewarding. Why is happiness important to business and workers?

One reason is that the stresses of the workplace is causing burnout and job transfers. A recent study showed 50% of the Millennials and 75% of the Generation Zers interviewed had left jobs because of stress and job dissatisfaction.

This is the age of job mobility. Whereas our forefathers were farmers or blacksmiths for life, younger workers are often changing jobs every three years. It is important for everyone to have a more comprehensive view of what makes them feel fulfilled, what enhances their workplace value, and how they can find better work life balance.

The importance for business and workers to discover the positive growth behaviors is that ignoring the right behaviors and seeking negative behaviors to relieve stress is what is killing us. Never before in the history of man has poor health and stress caused so much burn out, depression, drug abuse, and disillusionment.

In a newspaper article by Melissa Healy, she says "It's offic al. Americans are dying much earlier in life. The twin trends-an increased probability of death in midlife and a population-wide reversal of longevity-set the United States in stark contrast to every other affluent country in the world."

It is important for business to support workers in finding more satisfaction in their lives which will then promote their work life balance. The behaviors suggested in this Course aim at placing everyone on the path to greater learning, creativity, making bigger contributions to their circles, finding improved health, and getting fit.

These are the behaviors of growth and happiness. The reason I can say this with confidence is that science has proven that the right survival behaviors stimulate the happiness neurotransmitters and hormones of dopamine, serotonin, oxytocin, and endorphin. We can experience them every day and many times a day.

We can find positive and negative behaviors to stimulate a moment of happiness, but where we get in trouble is when the happiness stimulus is over, our brain defaults to cortisol, a stress hormone. We always have the choice of a positive or negative behavior.

What are the negative behaviors often pursued as a result of cortisol and stress? Cigarettes, sugar, caffeine, alcohol, overeating, drugs, pills, anger, shopping, gambling, and being sedentary, to name a few.

To gain the upper hand, we want to plan the positive behaviors in our schedule ahead of time. This is how we win. We want our positive behaviors to begin diminishing our desire for negative behaviors. We will learn about "keystone habits" that can change everything.

As we develop positive behaviors, the next experiences become career advancement, purpose, contribution, health, and fulfillment. As we pursue our negative behaviors the next experiences become depression, anxiety, obesity, cardiovascular disease, cancer, and chronic pain.

We don't need to chase so many fantasized dreams that often include possessions, money, power, and fame although each is a good goal. We can build happiness into our daily lives and maybe the fantasy will become different than we expected. We may learn the journey is the destination.

Chapter Two

What Are the Best Happiness Behaviors?

Let's look at what Nature would say if she didn't still consider us early man but could see the modern environment in which we live. We don't have to gather and hunt for food or join tribes to share workloads and provide protection.

We are in need of fulfilling careers, providing for our families, staying healthy, and having fun. How do we optimize our value and vitality so we are productive and live rich long lives? These are the kinds of goals Nature supports.

So, let's dig in. What are the behaviors?

<u>Learning</u>

Learning is challenge. With challenge, your brain creates more neurons and networks. There might not be a limit to how large your brain can grow, but we know by science that your brain shrinks with disuse as we get older. Disuse is a primary cause of dementia. Our brain has plasticity which means it can grow until we die.

What are the practices of learning? Studying material through reading, listening, visual aids. Taking classes that teach you new body movements. Improving or learning new skills and challenging material through any media, classes, mentorship, coaching, observation, or practice.

Learning is a survival opportunity that increases our ability to improve our lives and make a contribution. Both acts result in stimulating dopamine, serotonin, and oxytocin. Our best learning phases seem to peak as teenagers because we are accumulating and memorizing information on new topics. College extends the expansion of our ability to assimilate knowledge. But then what happens? We begin a career and often the work becomes the same every day. We stop growing.

Once we get the routines of careers, we rarely seek the challenge of learning new information, developing skills, being creative, and taking risks. These are the activities of growth scientists classify under the behavior of learning. These are the activities classified in Nature as survival opportunities. These are the activities Nature's has intended for you if you want predictable sustainable happiness. We think a BMW is happiness, but it is a by product of the right behaviors. It only makes us feel happy for a little while and then we need a new peak.

<u>Creativity</u>

Creativity is a personally unique or novel approach/engagement to solving problems, learning, or making art. Creativity is a process that is most effective with two steps. The first step is focus on a particular problem, art, science, skill, or process. The second important step is to have relaxation time when the information studied can incubate and organize within our subconscious for breakthroughs or epiphanies. Steven Kotler in *The Rise of Superman* said creativity is pattern recognition which leads to new innovations.

We can be creative in any endeavor. The difference between creativity and routine is routine doesn't require thinking or challenge. Creativity is exploration of an interest or problem to make something that doesn't exist. If I try to solve a problem, the successful solution will be something new. If I am writing a book, each page is something that didn't exist previously.

If I am working on new products, new services, or new processes in business that lead to greater sales, efficiency, or customer satisfaction, I am being creative. These are all survival opportunities that stimulate happiness and grow us.

Creativity is self-expression. Most anything we do is expressing us. The secret for happiness is to continuously work on expressing who we are by creating new work, ideas, or contributions. We get a happiness bonus if we plan to share to improve other lives.

Being an entrepreneur is being creative. Teaching can be creative when we are trying to find the best way to convey a message to our audience. Collaborating can be creative when engaged in group think to solve problems or develop something that doesn't exist.

Creativity sessions should be prioritized. Creativity should be at a time when our full brain is engaged because there are no interruptions. It can be time spent in work, art, hobbies, or for public service.

We can start planning creative time in our days to enhance our career opportunities. Who in business rises faster than those who are creative and often solve problems we didn't realize we had until we enjoy the new conveniences? Did we ever think we needed sticky notes, purchases delivered the same day, a phone with a camera or a car that drives itself?

<u>Contribution</u>

Contribution is sharing or caring. We are using our talents or time to affect other lives, processes, products, mankind, or the planet. It is a positive act to make things better.

In the acts of learning and creativity we improve our opportunity to contribute. Early man improved his hunting skills to bring more food to the community. Creating revenues through our skills or knowledge can affect lots of circles.

Contributing could be engaging in our own self-actualization which has the result of also improving everything around us. Self-actualization is connecting to who we are, what is possible, finding our purpose, feeling unity with all things, and optimizing our potential.

In this process of pursuing our potential, we gain the most humanistic emotions of empathy, compassion, and generosity. Learning to be empathetic is one of the brain's greater challenges. Emotional intelligence is certainly a survival enhancement.

Self-actualizing may seem selfish as we take personal time to discover who we are and become more than we were yesterday, but it is a generous act that will flow onto those around us and make life better for everyone. If everyone were self-actualizing, we would not have most of the problems we experience in the world today.

<u>Health and Fitness</u>

We are born with the capability of living robust, vital, and energized lives. The energy of children can be perpetuated with an obvious degree of modification as we mature. We have many behaviors that can improve health.

We can improve our nutrition, exercise, balance our emotions, and build spirituality. Each of these areas improve how we feel, how we perform, our ability to build our social status, and our desire to contribute to others.

The line between healthy and unhealthy can be the difference between feeling happy with our lives and feeling burdened by life. There is no fun in being overweight, constantly ill, having chronic pain, and experiencing the deterioration of all our physical capabilities.

The Ace Coaching Manual claims only 3% of Americans eat healthy, have an exercise routine, maintain a healthy weight and don't smoke. Certainly, we can raise that percentage in the workplace by adopting the right survival behaviors.

We have a responsibility to ourselves if we are to experience the glories of being alive. Health and fitness are spiritual experiences. They are an indication we are connected to our bodies, Nature, and the Universe. We can't ignore the rules followed by all living things on earth.

Healthy and fit people know that if you don't continuously take care of your body, it will let you down and doctors and pharmacies will become your lifeline. Healthy people want to avoid both doctors and medicine. They fear the intrusion of poor health on their ambitions. Consequently, fitness becomes a daily ritual that improves their days.

Sedentary people can begin with walking 10 to 15 minutes a day and aim for 150 minutes a week; that would be 30 minutes a day, five days a week. Add two days of resistance training at the gym and they are joining the world of the fit.

As a Health Coach and Personal Trainer, I have seen people turn their lives around in a short time by pledging to adopt some new behaviors. It starts with the first modification.

In the book *Younger Next Year*, Chris Crowley and Dr. Henry S. Lodge say there is no reason we cannot enjoy a high quality of life until we are 85 years old. Their prescription is an hour of exercise six days a week.

Chapter Three

What Are the Happiness and Stress Hormones and Neurotransmitters?

The happiness brain chemicals of dopamine, serotonin, oxytocin, and endorphin are stimulated when we are striving to reach our potential. Reaching our potential requires that we are continuously growing. Unfortunately, there is no rest in our striving if we want to continuously experience the happiness Nature provides.

Dopamine can be stimulated with the intentions of improving our survival opportunities and while we are engaged and focused. It might be our intention to write a book, take a course, eat healthy, start an exercise program, spend more time on teams at work, decide to solve a problem that has been plaguing us for years, or the intention to end bad behaviors. Dopamine is experienced when we are in "flow" to sustain our enjoyment of the activity. "Flow" is a focused state of engagement.

Serotonin occurs with lots of different activities. It is a reward chemical for achieving or making progress. When we feel proud of ourselves for an achievement or making a contribution, we get a serotonin boost. When we are in a good mood, serotonin is usually responsible. Any act of contribution, self-improvement, generosity, gratitude, charity, caring, or protecting is likely to generate serotonin and perks of happiness.

Oxytocin and serotonin can run together. Acts that contribute to the welfare of others and thereby lift our feelings about ourselves and raise our social status can stimulate oxytocin. It is the cuddle hormone so romance, family, and friends can all stimulate happiness from Nature's desire for us to form community.

Our desire to contribute at work for the benefit of co-workers, our company, our customers, or going green for the planet can all stimulate oxytocin. Developing skills that will serve the public like medicine, yoga, coaching, and teaching can stimulate oxytocin.

Endorphin is the hormone that reduces pain and converts maximum physical effort to pleasure. It is sometimes confused with anandamides which cross the brain barrier in runners high, but they work together.

Endorphin also stimulates serotonin, so while exercising and pushing our limits, we are feeling a euphoria. Early man was very physical. Our body needs the inflammation flushing from exercise and the muscle building from exertion to flourish. All the benefits to our brain, cardiovascular health, immunity, and emotional balance are maintained by exercising our body and pushing our limits. Everything that stimulates endorphin is building our survival opportunities.

The flip side of happiness chemicals are the stress hormones which act to protect us and induce us to find happiness in more survival behaviors. Yes, the brain is continuously pushing us to find happiness because happiness is survival.

Stress hormones indicate we are in danger or worrying about a problem. Early man responded by solving each situation. Today, we respond with too many behaviors that are self-destructive.

This is why boredom, the "to do lists", the emails, the urgent unimportant activities, and the mindless activities like surfing the web, keep us immersed in cortisol and negative growth instead of feeling the pleasures of positive behaviors and positive growth. Our brain defaults to cortisol pretty quickly after we have experienced happiness. This is meant to induce us to solve the next problem.

In early man it often meant searching for the next meal. In modern man it might be looking for work solutions, or learning something to increase our employment value. It could be working on something that will benefit others. Solving problems might mean improving the welfare of our family, friends, and the community at large.

Adrenaline and norepinephrine are the action stress hormones that can enhance physical performance in times of threat or to excel in necessary physical feats. When these hormones are activated, some systems shut down and others are expanded. In exercising or sports, adrenaline can enhance performance. If we stimulate adrenaline worrying about problems, we are causing physical harm. We obviously don't want to remain in heightened states of alarm or fear for long periods of time.

Chapter Four

Why Do We Move from Happiness to Stress?

As stated before, in Nature's scheme, we are still early man. She doesn't realize we have all these labor-saving devices. Homo sapiens is 30,000 years old and life began 3 billion years ago. Modern man is a blip in time. Our systems have not evolved to any great degree out of the survival of the fittest mentality. Our systems still think dangers lurk and survival is difficult. Regardless of our station in life, we still worry every day.

We don't often think we are worried about survival, but our organism is totally in survival mode. When we cut back on calories to lose weight, our metabolism slows because our body thinks its winter and we can't find food. Regardless of how much we own, we are aware of economic, competitive, and political issues that could affect our wellbeing. The rich are just as worried as everyone else otherwise there wouldn't be lobbyists and political contributions.

When we are not engaged in survival opportunities that stimulate happiness, our brain immediately defaults to cortisol which causes us to worry. The brain says you just got promoted, but now you have more responsibility and there are expectations. You won the Super Bowl, but what about next year? You just had a beautiful baby, but now you have to be a great parent.

The struggle for survival continues every day in our bodies and brain. The way we reduce cortisol is to have enough growth activities that promise our struggle will be minimized. If we are proactive and plan the growth activities into our days, we are automatically reducing the duration of the cortisol.

Where the big physical and mental health issues arise are when the stress hormones push people to negative behaviors for relief. Instead of a positive behavior people pick the next available solution. These solutions can be quick. Sugar, eating, alcohol, drugs, pills, and shopping bring easy relief.

Worrying is a mental act and anxiety is a full body engagement. Worry is the alert that something needs to be fixed and not an alarm of overwhelming danger. When we are anxious, it should be about life and death situations. We have few of those, but in modern times, job security is the substitute.

We are frequently anxious about dangers that have a slim chance of occurring. Anxiety shuts down digestion, immunity and blood flow to certain parts of the body not important in emergencies. It is meant to occur for just a short period of time and then be resolved.

When something worries us, it is time to make a positive plan. It might be an opportunity to schedule creative time. Nothing fixes problems like creativity. It is important to distinguish from the real dangers posed and not let our-selves get taken down roads that are not necessary.

When we have positive behaviors scheduled into our day that may include action or may just be solitude, we can look ahead from our anxious moment to the relief coming soon in a positive behavior. If I am worried about a project, but know I have a break or am going to the gym in an hour, it becomes a support for our emotional health.

We want to stay in the calmer states of beta brain waves or creative and meditative states of alpha and theta waves. Alpha and theta waves run between 7 hertz and 12 hertz. Beta waves run to 30 hertz. Over 30 hertz we are experiencing gamma brain waves and our body shifts to a long list of reactions that prepare us for maximum response. Gamma rays for a lizard come before attacking for food or running from a predator.

Thinking we can find a solution will calm our nervous system. When we don't think we have a solution, we remain in the fear/high anxiety mode. Our brain is constantly measuring our wellness and looking for danger. It subconsciously evaluates all our systems such as breathing, heart rate, digestion, circulation, sugar levels, caffeine, and alcohol.

Our senses are constantly aware of threats. When the senses pick up an external threat, our brain puts us on alert. Our systems are so hyper aware that if something is flying at our head, we will duck before we think.

In more slow-moving threats, the danger is raised, but then the prefrontal cortex evaluates the threat and judges whether we can deal with it. The reason military personnel practice is so that danger becomes recognizable and our reactions are rationale and effective.

We can habituate to danger to the point it becomes familiar. We praise professional athletes for being cool, calm, and collected. In extreme sports, athletes are confident they have the skills to face the life-threatening dangers.

They drop into "flow" immediately where they are no longer thinking but rely on their total brain and intuition to react faster than thought. They experience dopamine, endorphin, anandamides, serotonin, and adrenaline. In their words they are experiencing "pure bliss" and unity with all things. Adrenaline junkies are going for the feelings.

In our daily lives, we can become aware of our worrying and know we can solve these thoughts with positive resolutions. We can become habituated to dealing with everyday challenges from the confidence we have faced these problems before and triumphed.

Entrepreneurs say they jump from the airplane and then put on their parachutes because they are comfortable and enjoy challenges. They have become habituated to facing the unknown and triumphing. We can develop confidence in our skills to prevail.

To enjoy more energizing feelings, we can take more risks and get out of our comfort zones. Risks don't have to be to our mortality, but they can be slightly above our current skills and push toward growing us.

We move from worry to happiness as we face problems and solve them. We are getting a big dose of happiness chemicals when we struggle with problems and make progress. We should be continuously looking for survival opportunities (ways to grow). We could be in a continuous state of happiness. This makes life exciting and fulfilling. We have too much non-productive time that is boring and stressful. We should have as many positive behaviors in our lives as possible each day.

Chapter Five

What Are Keystone Habits?

A "keystone habit" described by Charles Duigg in the *The Power of Habit* is one good habit that may change all of our habits.

From *The Power of Habit*:

"When people start habitually exercising, even as infrequently as once a week, they start changing other unrelated patterns in their lives, often unknowingly. Typically, people who exercise start eating better and becoming more productive at work. They smoke less and show more patience with colleagues and family. They use their credit cards less and say they feel less stressed. It's not completely clear why. But for many people exercise is a keystone habit that triggers widespread change."

In another example from *The Power of Habit* about how will-power can result in changing all our habits one at a time:

"Oaten and Cheng did one more experiment. They enrolled forty-five students in an academic improvement program that focused on creating study habits. Predictably, students learning skills improved. And the students also smoked less, drank less, watched less television, exercised more, and ate healthier, even though all those things were never mentioned in the academic program."

I found that focusing on eating better foods to lose 50 pounds many years ago led to new fitness routines, a stronger feeling of connection to all things, a desire to contribute by writing blogs on fitness, health, and spirituality, the loss of the 50 pounds, and an entirely new way of eating. The desire to contribute so others would feel better led to my desire to do more coaching. The eating habit not only changed my weight, but the thrust of my life.

What are some behaviors you would like to change? What are some healthy alternatives you could adapt into your daily schedule or negative behaviors you could drop? The most basic change can change everything.

Adding a learning, creativity, or an exercise block into your routine every day could change everything. As you begin to make progress, it is only natural to wonder what else you could do to improve your wellbeing.

Chapter Six

You Have More Time Than You Think

Our schedules seem crowded, but not all the activities are valuable. When I was in real estate, a guru named Doug Yeaman was conducting training for the real estate industry. In the first session he asked us to track the time spent in our activities for a week. At the end of the week, he wanted us to categorize them as productive, indirectly productive, or non-productive.

For real estate, productive was working on listings or with buyers. Indirectly productive time was soliciting for listings or working to get buyers. Everything else was non-productive. Non-productive included paperwork, meetings, "to do lists', and distractions.

At the end of the week, I found 64% of my time was non-productive. Yeaman said with so much non-productive time, we could instead take a day off or engage in an activity we thought we didn't have time for. In the long run, missing non-productive activities wouldn't have any effect on our productivity.

We're held hostage by our schedules and "to do lists" and think we don't have the time for purposeful activities. Try tracking your activities for a week and see how many activities are important. Sometimes urgent and non-important have too much time on our schedule and we certainly fill our days with distractions and non-important activities such as social media, surfing the internet, endless email, TV, and negative habits for relief.

Chapter Seven

Building Productivity

Some of our most important drivers have been categorized by Daniel Pink in *Drive: The Surprising Truth About What Motivates Us*":

"Human beings have an innate inner drive to be autonomous, self-determined, and connected to one another. And when that drive is liberated, people achieve more and live richer lives."

These drives are happiness chemical stimulators. It's no wonder our strongest drives result in our happiest or most contented feelings. Being autonomous, self-determined (Maslow said Self-Actuated), and connected, we are stimulating dopamine, serotonin, and oxytocin. We stimulate them because we are experiencing high level survival opportunities.

We can be entrepreneurial in our days when we learn or work on solutions for our work. We can be driven to find answers our company or our customers are seeking. Think of the creative efforts being exerted daily at Amazon, Apple, Google and Tesla. There are races to be the first for the best solutions and services that will lead the market.

Look for the opportunities to engage in activities that are cutting edge and will solve problems for our co-workers, employers, customers, stake holders, and the community at large. All the happiness brain chemicals are awaiting in this search.

We might have to learn and engage in creative time. These are the indirect activities that lead to the productive activities. Writing a book, finding business solutions, inventing devices, and researching are all good examples of engaging in these drives.

The more time we spend in building our value and thinking of the contribution to a larger circle, the more happiness chemicals we are experiencing. Leaving the tedium and time wasting or stressful activities to a minimum is reducing our cortisol and stress.

The more time we spend in positive activities the fewer negative habits we are likely to continue. If we can develop a thrust for improvement of our bodies, minds, souls, and workplace issues, we are on a happiness path.

We need to have something that gets us up in the morning. We want to build a list of positive behaviors from learning and creativity to exercise, rest, and recovery. Many people are out doing bike rides, surfing, running or going to the gym in the mornings.

Workers with less time can do exercises in their home to start their day. They can do yoga or just stretch, lift some dumbbells, follow an exercise video, jump on a treadmill, stationary bike or stair master, meditate or just sit in solitude gathering strength for the upcoming day.

Creativity needs a fresh nervous system. I am most creative in the morning and after an exercise session or after an afternoon "time out'. Don't think of it as a waste of time, but as a break to rebuild your creative energy. We should try to operate at our peak as often as possible.

Start scrutinizing the activities, people, meetings, "to do lists", distractions, and negative habits that rob your energy and leave you feeling worse than when you started. Maybe organize all these time wasters into one block.

I can be in flow in the morning, mid- afternoon and evenings from taking the right "time outs". I am not worn out at night, I am usually energized and satisfied that I made progress during the day with the habits and behaviors that are part of my long-term goals.

You might be saying "I don't have any of those opportunities". "I don't have the time." "I have too many obligations". "I have too much responsibility". "I have too much pressure".

I know you have all these responses. I am a coach. The purpose of the Course is to start considering how you would like your day compared to perhaps how it is.

Your life can develop a sort of muscle memory from routines and patterns of thinking that don't serve your happiness. Injecting more positive experiences into your day will necessitate creating some positive habits. You might not be used to this. You might struggle and want to go back to your old ways.

Maybe you don't want more happiness in your days. We do get a certain pleasure in doting on our unhappiness as proof the world is a bad place. The brain actually reinforces this thinking. We might have developed neural pathways that are cynical and pessimistic. Living with negative thoughts actually can produce dopamine and serotonin if we are convinced we are right and find evidence every day to support this thinking.

Chapter Eight

Cognitive Therapy

Cognitive Therapy has become an essential element of coaching because we are challenged to move people from negative beliefs to positive beliefs. The only way people make this transition is by engaging in new behaviors and discovering they love them.

When someone talks to me about losing weight or getting in shape or changing their life, there is usually a history of failed attempts and preconceived notions of failure; there are always obstacles. Time is always a major hindrance and "responsibilities" are next in line. Lacking support from mates, family, or work can greatly interfere with a desired goal.

The next major obstacle and challenge for clients and coaches to reaching their goals is relapse. This is the stage where people decide the changes are too difficult and emotionally challenging. They decide it was much more comfortable to live with their problems than move to a more promising solution.

Let's do the exercises included in this course to air out the notions and beliefs we are living with that may be imprisoning us. First, we have to acknowledge where we are. Then we think about how we would like things to be. Then we create starting strategies. Once engaged, we can reach a status coaches call self-efficacy where the rewards become the motivation.

There are big budgets being spent for "Well Being" to make workers' lives different. Someone cares. Business needs your help in deciding whether and how to budget support. It is to their benefit that you become more productive and happier. With the modernization of business using AI and robots, businesses need workers to be more vital and committed. If there are going to be fewer workers, as some fear, they will have to be the best workers.

If you take the suggestions of this Course and start creating new perspectives, you might find that you can better articulate your needs and improve your communications at work in seeking support.

Creating goals and having someone support your progress is a path to self-efficacy in which you no longer need support but are self-motivating.

Chapter Nine

Increase Productivity by Creating Blocks of Time

"During a peak experience," Maslow explained, 'the individual experiences an expansion of self, a sense of unity, and meaningfulness in life. The experience lingers in one's consciousness and gives a sense of purpose, integration, self-determination and empathy.' These states, he concluded, were the hidden commonality among all high achievers, the source code of intrinsic motivation:" Steven Kotler *The Rise of Superman*

One of the most effective ways to creating happiness brain chemicals, being more productive and feeling satisfaction from our activities is to put our activities in blocks of time.

Interruptions in our activities make it more difficult to get into "flow". While in "flow", our brain produces dopamine to sustain our level of effort. Dopamine helps us match patterns. It promotes epiphanies. Athletes have been known to perform moves they had never tried before just because the situation demanded it and their subconscious recognized the need. Extreme athletes get to "flow" immediately to stay alive. They need their awareness to be faster than their thinking.

Athletes, speakers, and artists certainly understand how getting into "flow" improves focus and performance. It is a state when all our systems operate in synchronicity and reduce (eliminate) conflicting thoughts and negativity. As I mentioned earlier, flow shuts down the prefrontal cortex from which judgements and criticism arise. If we are speaking in front of an audience, we want our most positive self to be in control.

I am fortunate to be able to create blocks of time in my day where I have few interruptions. I have exercise blocks, time for writing, teaching by appointment blocks, learning blocks, and leisure blocks. I can literally flow from one activity to the next and perform at peak in each block. At the end of the day I have usually maximized my capabilities and enjoyment in each block. I go for flow because it optimizes my time.

At the end of the day, I can quantify what I have achieved. I could journal what I achieved in each block. I do journal my exercise and I summarize my week in an email or a phone call with my support partner on Fridays. He also reports on his week and, as friends, we exchange new developments, what our kids are doing, and what we are working on.

In many workers' lives, interruptions are the norm. This can keep us in states of hyper alert and stress our nervous system. When we cannot focus on an activity, we cannot deliver our best capabilities. Sometimes this is built into a job position. We are expected to produce while accepting interruptions.

If we had choice, we might schedule our days differently. At the end of the day we might feel more accomplished and satisfied if we were able to deliver our best in each time block.

What times would you like to assign to each of these activities?

Productivity (9 a.m. to 4 p.m.)

Exercise (7 a.m. to 8 a.m.) (4:30 p.m. to 6 p.m.)

Creativity (9 a.m. to 10:30 a.m.)

Rest break (1 p.m. to 1:30 p.m.)

Leisure activities (6 p.m. to 9 p.m.)

Socializing (6 p.m. to 9 p.m.)

Learning (5 a.m. to 6 a.m.) (8 p.m. to 9 p.m.)

Hobbies (6 p.m. to 9 p.m.)

You might be saying I don't have time for half of these activities. A good start is recognizing what could be in your days that is not. These are the activities we want to include to have fulfilling days. Being fulfilled is likely to make you more productive and operating at 100% instead of feeling burnt out and operating at 50%. I usually get 6 out of 8 of these activities in my day.

The next step would be to schedule our most important blocks to our highest periods of energy. I am best in the morning, but exercise during the day creates my next best block. Effective "time outs" which sometimes is a 20-minute nap creates another premium time block.

When are your recovery breaks? Recovery is the secret to more productivity. Recovery is relaxation which rests our nervous system and refreshes us. It is a reset. Recovery sets up our next productivity block.

What are some time blocks you could allocate to recovery and relaxation? We need not feel guilty about doing nothing. Warren Buffet said this is intelligent behavior.

Exercise	Hours	__________________
Meditation	Hours	__________________
Nap	Hours	__________________
Walk	Hours	__________________
Music	Hours	__________________
Solitude	Hours	__________________
Socializing	Hours	__________________
Family Time	Hours	__________________

Look at creating your most effective time blocks for the most important activities. First you would decide what you would include in each time block. Maybe you would start including things not in your life right now. Most of these time blocks would create happiness brain chemicals because you would probably get into "flow" with this uninterrupted time.

Maybe you would find new passions or include passions that you now have no time to express. This is your life and you want to make it the life of your dreams. Everyone around you would benefit if you could make it happen. Look for the support.

Chapter Ten

Procrastination

Procrastination is an energy killer. We worry. We fail to engage. We become overwhelmed as deadlines approach. Procrastinators often need the stress of a deadline to get moving. It has been said that people with ADHD need pressure to begin an assignment or project.

Starting everything early, on the other hand, is an energy builder. We have the luxury of time to do our best work. We build self-esteem. We're done by the deadline. There is great satisfaction in completing things early. It becomes an attitude and way of life.

Conquering procrastination could be a game changer for productivity. You start looking further ahead to what might help your career and create more resilience. The best way to beat the competition is to keep reinventing yourself.

Name things on which you procrastinate.

Work deadlines   ____

Getting to appointments   ____

Buying gifts   ____

Paying bills   ____

Calling people   ____

Getting exercise   ____

Other   ____

As a whole, people fall into two groups-procrastinators and non-procrastinators. It's like people who are late vs people who are early. They are related. If you are a procrastinator or a late bird, what are your beliefs that support this habit(s)? What would have to happen for you to decide that starting early and/or arriving on time is important?

Along these lines, what are some of the things you would like to see in your future that you have been putting off?

- Taking a course
- Learning something interesting or career oriented
- Taking a vacation
- Spending more time with family
- Starting an exercise program
- Eating better

Anything you could start today?

Consider, the longer you engage in something daily, the easier it gets. Therefore, the sooner you start and make it a regular practice, the less you will have to worry about finding the motivation to engage.

What are some of the things you could engage in each day that would deliver some great results in the future? Physical exercise is easy to increase once engaged for a few weeks. I built push-ups from 10 to 70 by doing one more each day. I built my bike rides from 11 miles to 40 miles from engaging several times a week.

While I am doing my bike rides after I wake up, I am hardly thinking about the bike ride anymore. My mind is somewhere else while I am riding as I let my mind wander and maintain consciousness of the safety around me. I am appreciating how beautiful it is in the early mornings riding along the coast and glad I am out before most people are on the road. When I am done, I have completed something that is now an important part of my life.

Pick something that will become easier as you engage and make it important in your life. It becomes an important contributor to your daily happiness.

What's first?

1>

Think of something you would like to do or accomplish, but starting scares or terrifies you? You have been procrastinating for a long time? Or maybe it's on your bucket list and you would love to check it off.

What kind of information, skills, mentoring, tutoring, conditioning, or financing would be a first step?

Who could help or be a support?

- Mate
- Parents
- Boss
- School Counselor

My friend, at 70 years old, wanted to climb to Mt. Everest base camp at 17,500 feet. He was not in shape. He started with 4-mile walks and conditioned for a year. He made it. The first step is the important one.

What would be the first step you could take in a new goal?

1>

Fear is something overwhelming to your perceived capabilities. Taking one bite at a time makes the fear smaller. If I want to surf 8' waves, I have to start with 2' waves.

What is something you fear but want to do?

1>

What would be the first bite? A lesson? A Coach? YouTube? A book? A course? Or just jump in?

1>

How will you feel in the future if you never tried to do something that was a dream?

The main difference between those who accomplish great things and those who stay stuck is that first step.

What is the biggest fear holding you back?

- Injury
- Fear of failure
- Criticism from others
- Steep learning curve
- Your own internal voice saying you can't do it
- Financial
- Competition
- Past failures
- Time

Chapter Eleven

Relapse

The real obstacle to meaningful change is relapse. This is what occurs when you decide that the new habits are too painful and that the old habits would be more comfortable even if they may mean misery. We love routine and familiarity. We will endure lots of pain rather than seek a new process.

When health coaches train new people, the first cause of relapse is usually caused by the obstacle of "time". The second cause of relapses is taking a vacation from the routine like binging at a party or for a weekend. We have to build in the possibility of relapses and be committed to get back on track.

Progress to new goals requires we leave our comfort zones and become someone new. Our identity will change as we go from obese to lean, sedentary to fit, a beginner to a master, a follower to a leader, poor to rich, unknown to an authority, and depressed to happy.

The health industry finds that at least 50% of people can't make the transition. It would be the same in other types of endeavors. We don't like change, but it is the bridge to the promised land. It takes courage. We have to face our fears and our preconceptions and our misconceptions. It is rarely worse on the other side of the bridge. It is usually better. You have to be wiling to accept the new "you".

Relapse is like crawling out of a hole to see the sunshine and deciding it is too bright. It is refusing to accept our destiny. It is unwillingness to test our potential. It is missing what creates happiness. Growth is the happiness trail.

Can you pick an area for growth that might become a "keystone habit" and result in you being someone you are not today?

Can you get someone to share your effort and support you?

Who? ______________

Can you write out a plan or strategy?

Could you do something every day that would get you closer to making the first move?

Often your early difficulties and how you overcame the initial resistance and then met challenges is a process others would enjoy hearing. It is the central theme of many movies and books and often songs. The heroes always have a challenge.

In one of Tom Cruise's *Mission Impossible* movies, he told his handler, Anthony Hopkins, that the assignment would be more than difficult. Anthony Hopkins replied "Of course, that's why we don't call it Mission Difficult."

Visualization is a powerful process and used by many coaches for professional athletes. In studies, the difference between those who engaged in live practices like shooting baskets and those who visualized the results were often very close in final testing.

There is always some way others would benefit in you sharing how you got the courage to start and how you learned. Would you be willing to share your path? Facebook and Instagram are story books. Your brain stimulates oxytocin in the process of you sharing something that could help others. Bloggers are addicted to the self-expression, the thought of helping, and the rewarding feedback.

Make a goal of journaling your personal story each week. Knowing you have to write something each week gives you a guide to what's next. Share your progress with someone else who could be your support team. Could you start journaling this week? Start talking about what scares you at this moment. I have traded weekly reports with a friend for over ten years. We both value the exchange and never miss.

Dan Briton wrote a book called *One Word*. It is the one word that might be your purpose or reason for being here. Actor, musician, store owner, chef, runner, physicist, doctor, writer, CEO, marketing guru, or hiker? Think of people and see if you attach a one word to their image. Taylor Swift? Tom Brady? Warren Buffet?

Do you have a one word?

1>

When you start on a path that becomes a passion and then feels like your purpose, it might become your one word. I certainly think of myself as bike rider, surfer, surf coach, lifestyle coach, writer, reader, amateur chef, gym rat, and father.

Have several.

Chapter Twelve

Our Addiction to Speed

We have an addiction to speed and producers of goods and services are bent on feeding that addiction. You can now get products you buy online the next day and often the same day. If you contact someone by phone or online, you expect an answer in a few hours. Internet speed is continuously increasing and Google downgrades websites that don't light up in two seconds.

Are we making ourselves crazy? I love speed. I expect speed. Yet, we have to consider how our nervous systems deal with slow. How do we feel when traffic becomes stalled? How do we feel when things don't arrive on time? What happens when people don't respond to us right away? How do we feel about any slow service? We have existed with slow in the past. Before we had email, we had letter openers. Vacations are supposed to return us to "the slow" for a week.

How fast do we expect to progress in our careers? How much time do we give our current employer to promote or educate us? A lot of millennials are now changing jobs every two to three years because they are in a hurry to advance. Are we giving ourselves and processes enough time to show results?

As a surfing coach, I see new surfers rushing out to buy short boards before they know how to ride an easy board. They want to be like the experts they see in the movies but under-estimate the need to follow the steps. My boy students are frequently frustrated when they can't do something instantly. They have expectations that their abilities will deliver without having to learn the fundamentals.

We have to adjust our nervous systems to the fact some worthwhile accomplishments will take time and dedication. I go the gym every other day. I get stronger, but seeing physical results is difficult. It takes faith in the process and love of the process. I have faith the practice is good for me and can feel the difference in my body. My commitment is to go every other day and let the results speak for themselves. Patience is required.

How about our lives? How many long-term projects are we working on?

Specifically, we need long term outlooks on:

- Health
- Fitness
- Learning
- Relationships
- Skill development
- Careers

Allowing short term pressure, deadlines, and failure to see quick results can interfere with our learning process and can have long term detrimental effects.

Sometimes the long-term process is interrupted by the short-term focus on the time value of money. How much income is needed to meet the next outlay for expenses? Startups are continuously feeling the need to raise capital as operating expenses are greater than revenues. They try not to lose focus of their goals as they try to show promising short-term results.

Our families have time values for money as certain obligations need to be met regularly. This pressure increases with the need for normal childhood expenses like braces, school tuitions, clothes, lessons, and so on. We place time pressure on our children. How many activities do we squeeze in a week for them feeling they need to have great resumes starting now?

We have to be aware that depression and suicide thoughts are rampant in kids from the expectations they are facing. College students suffer from depression even though studying for advanced degrees. The graduates often grab the first job instead of looking for the right job and begin on the wrong course instead of the dream course. Short term expectations can rob us of the happiness we deserve.

The problem with time pressure is it interrupts flow, defers important long-term growth to feed short term deadlines, creates impatience and frustration, and, of course, all this results in stress.

Stress prevents happiness brain chemicals. If our lives are focused on speed and neglect long-term goals, we become focused on making all the short-term deadlines. We will be living at the effect of stress hormones instead of creating positive behaviors that deliver short and long term happiness.

We should have a perspective on which goals will take time and dedicate ourselves to preparing and taking the right steps. We should ask ourselves if we love the engagement enough to keep us going for the long haul. Is the result valuable enough to keep us committed until the goal is reached?

What do we need to get started? What do we need along the way? Who will support us in the process? How will we measure our progress? If we don't reach our goal, will we have been happy with what we did achieve or the fact we tried?

A few years ago, I wanted to ride my bike 100 miles in an annual event. I realized after a while that I didn't have the time to prepare and that I was already too late in getting started. I rode 70 miles in my work outs and was satisfied that for this goal, I had reached my limit. As I ride now, 70 miles remains my peak achievement. There is often a need to reset goals to reality. It doesn't make us a failure.

The practice of continuing to set goals is important. Each effort will grow us. I achieve happiness brain chemicals in my continuous efforts because I continue to achieve and enjoy the engagement. If I eventually ride 100 miles, I will be proud of my dedication. Yet, I was proud as I progressed to ride 30 and then 40 miles. After my 50-mile ride, I went to Stone Brewery and celebrated with a craft beer. The journey is as important if not more so than the destination.

Other practices require time and patience. We should become aware that we need some time each day to exercise and maintain our health. We need "time outs" each day to level our nervous systems. We need time with our families before our kids are grown. We need time in our lives to enjoy the current moment or after a while our lives become a blur.

I learn at every opportunity and will find time to read or study. I make writing a priority which is beneficial to my career but is also a time when I am fully engaged without interruption. I feel each few years I am a better writer. Writing takes time and I may never be great, but I will be better. I am always happy writing. Engaging in our passions is autotelic meaning the activity is the reward.

Creativity, learning, health, fitness, and contribution all need uninterrupted time. They are essential to our growth and wellbeing. They create happiness brain chemicals and the purpose and reasons we enjoy life. They may lead to quicker prosperity because they grow our value. They may not happen quickly, but day by day they do evolve. All five together create a great journey.

Chapter Thirteen

The Narrative Self and Experiencing Self

Yuval Harari in his book *Home Deus* spelled out how we all experience the narrative self vs the experiencing self. The narrative self makes New Year's Resolutions. The experiencing-self interferes when it's time to put on your running shoes or not eat the chocolate cake.

Name some of the things you have pledged to do and then stopped when it came time to execute?

How many things have you pledged <u>not</u> to do but did anyway when the temptation or stimulus or boredom was there? How many people in the world are trying to lose 10 pounds and never achieve it?

Doug Yeaman said you knew a commitment by the result. If you didn't get the result, you were not committed. He said by example, how committed are you to get to the airport on time for a vacation? Think about something you didn't accomplish because you gave up.

We get stopped by the obstacles. The beauty of passions is they don't allow obstacles to be more than a bump. Commitment also gets us through obstacles. I like Yeaman's metaphor that every wall has a door. With passions we don't worry about failure because our main motivation is to engage.

The engagement takes us to our destinations even if we don't know where that will be. A person who loves playing the violin never knows if they will be

great. They just keep playing for the love of it. Did
Wayne Gretsky know he would be great as he
practiced at five years old? Did Bill Gates envision
Microsoft as he was writing a single line of code
on a card and pushing it into the early computers?
Did Warren Buffet know what would happen as he
looked for value in companies? Investment in a
shingle share of his stock years ago at $8,000
would be worth several hundred thousand dollars
now.

If I am committed to climbing a specific mountain, I
will know I was committed by the result. If I am
committed to writing a book, I will know I was
committed by the result. If I want to be President
of a company, I won't know the result before I
invest years of effort.

Chapter Fourteen

Combining Our Behaviors

This course has covered five basic growth activities to achieve daily happiness: learning, creating, contributing, health, and fitness.

What do we want to include in our daily activities?

- Learning challenging information or movement
- Creating something that expresses ourselves
- Making efforts to make our circles better
- Improving our health
- Getting our bodies in better physical condition

Stringing them together in a day creates a steady stream of happiness as we become better versions of ourselves on a daily basis. We are going to have dopamine for our intentions, serotonin from our achievements, and oxytocin for the benefits we are providing.

The stress hormones we might experience on a daily basis will have to fight for room in our brain. When the negative emotions occur in our schedule, they will be soon replaced by something more positive. Five positive activities a day should prevent negative emotions from dominating our emotions or becoming chronic. We might be able to substitute the positive activities to interrupt our down periods instead of some of the negative habits we have adopted. The more negative habits we can eliminate the easier it is to remain in a positive mental framework.

People often resist written plans more than they resist getting started with new practices. If you don't write down plans in advance, which would probably stimulate dopamine, it is motivating to write down accomplishments after the fact. It is an "I did it" that stimulates serotonin. It is fun to make a summary of a new interest on a daily basis to track progress.

I love to keep track of my exercise. In a monthly view calendar, I keep track of each bike ride with the time, distance and average speed. I keep track of each day I visit the gym. In the gym, I write down my exercises and sets, reps and weight. I can look at my workouts in a glance and see how much progress I am making.

As I bike, my average speed increases on a regular basis. As I lift weights, the amount I can lift increases. As I write or post, I am increasing my influence on the internet or adding pages to a book.

Progress in an interest makes it more addictive and easier to engage each time. I don't encounter resistance engaging in my activities because over time they have just become natural extensions of myself. The times I engage are usually the same each day so I just hop to it. They have become who I am.

Hopefully, this Life Style Self-Coaching Course will help you find your interests and create a map for building on your skills and passions. If you don't have passions, learning a skill can create a passion.

Many new surf students fall in love with it on their first session. For them, it could be a "lever" to getting in better shape, learning more about surfing, planning more ocean vacations, and moving to the beach. Starting new things can lead to passions. I love it when after a surf lesson(s), students say they are going to rent a surfboard the next day or want to move to San Diego for college.

Do you have an interest in growing? Do you have an interest in helping others grow? Do you have an interest in working with other people in a common mission, like your work? Do you have an interest in helping customers you serve have a better experience?

A lifestyle is how you live and what you do. Making choices to grow and help others grow are lifestyle values. I say fitness is a lifestyle. I say happiness is a lifestyle. People engaged in fitness often have it as a center for how they live. Health is the same. Some people would say music is their lifestyle. Others love work. Some live for families and their friends.

We can build on any passion. What is our passion taken to the next step? Do we want to become more accomplished, share more, or help others follow in our footsteps? Do we want to create something that serves the masses?

Engage in your passion. Find followers who love what you do and are extra supportive because you help a cause. This is why many companies go green or find worthwhile endeavors to support.

The public supports those causes with their purchasing power. Richard Branson insists each of his 300 companies have a community cause to support.

Mankind needs enlightened individuals and businesses.

Chapter Fifteen

Risk Taking

One of the most productive ways to encourage growth is by taking risks. Risks don't have to lead to our mortality. We can leave that to the extreme athletes. We can take everyday risks that promise to move us from the status quo to something more.

On a scale of one to ten, risks can be from leaving our comfort zone to engaging in something that threatens our mortality. Public speaking is a great growth exercise that creates fear in many people. Extreme athletes who rock climb, ski, jump, surf, and many other sports risk their mortality for the feelings. They believe we have unlimited capabilities and we can push until we find our limits.

When we compare the lives we lead with those of extreme athletes, we might wonder why we don't have more courage. Why don't we test who we are and find the feelings enjoyed by the extreme athletes? What are the feelings? They immediately enter "flow" in which their prefrontal cortex shuts down (criticism and self-judgement) and their full brain and body coordinate to move in some natural setting without fear. All the happiness brain chemicals are stimulated. They experience bliss.

When we leave our comfort zone to learn, create, exercise, engage socially, start a business, or work on a new project, we create vulnerabilities. In the vulnerabilities we are testing our ability to meet the challenge. This is where we find out who we are. It is difficult and scary at the start. Usually we find with consistent engagement that we are capable of meeting the challenge and then we start craving it. We might fear public speaking, entertaining an audience, assuming leadership, attempting a new skill, or cooking for the in laws.

While we are engaged, the question running through our mind, at first, is whether we can do it. Once we do it several times, we gain confidence and soon we are entering "flow" when we engage. "Flow" is the peak learning and creativity state because in shutting down the judgmental and critical prefrontal cortex, we are unleashing intuition, instinct, and the Universal Intelligence that guides peak performances.

Read *The Rise of Superman* in which Steven Kotler explores the motivation of extreme athletes and why they engage in mortality defying feats. If we want to move forward in our careers and personal lives, we might have to leave our comfort zones and bring our uniqueness to the task of expanding our talents. We are not made from cookie cutters. We are each extremely unique and the excitement in life is often finding the "how" we are unique.

Chapter Sixteen

Are you Prepared to Move Forward?

Three of Life's Choices from David Berry in *A More Daring Life*:

> *"One of three things is true:*
>
> 1. *You've got what you need to get started and you are afraid that it's insufficient for what the world expects.*
> 2. *You know what you need to get started-new information, skills, relationships-and now you've got to get it.*
> 3. *You don't know what you need because you don't know what you want.*
>
> *You either need to get moving, get learning or get clear. If only there were another way."*

This is a good time to stop and consider which of these three is relevant to you.

In our work and in our lives, we have reached certain states. There are things we would like to learn for work and things we would like to learn in our personal lives. Are we fully prepared with all the information and skills necessary to advance to the next step and only procrastination is holding us back? This might be the time for risk taking and moving forward with a plan.

Do we know what we need to learn, the skills we need to develop, or the relationships we need to form and just have not made the first step? This is the best time to start moving forward and obtaining the missing pieces we need for our plan.

Do we have no idea what we want or how we got to where we are? Sometimes this occurs when we graduate college and take the first job instead of finding what really resonates with our soul. In the middle of our careers we are wondering how we find something that would seem meaningful. This is a good time to take an assessment and decide what makes us get up in the morning and what we would love to be doing in our days. We might have to start learning and exploring to find a passion(s). Once we have a passion, the road opens and what we want to do is no longer a mystery.

We can spend a lot of our days just fulfilling our obligations not directing our attention to specific goals. We should have at least four or five practices bent on improvement that will all result in us having more success and fulfillment. Consistency and commitment to our activities is important. Engaging in the five behaviors of this course can become your passion as you find you are moving forward in your career and personal life and discovering what makes you happy.

COURSE QUESTIONS

As you progress through questions don't feel limited by the three slots provided for answers. Feel free to add paper and create more answers or make them longer.

What are some practices you could begin now to build the 5 behaviors covered in this Course?

Learning

1>____________________________________

2> ____________________________________

3>____________________________________

Creativity

1>____________________________________

2>____________________________________

3>____________________________________

Contribution

1>____________________________________

2>____________________________________

3>____________________________________

Health

1>____________________________________

2>____________________________________

3>____________________________________

Fitness

1>____

2>____

3>____

Could you start your day with exercise or creativity? You would be building happiness brain chemicals with each, building your survival opportunities, increasing your vitality, improving your ability to contribute, and building resilience for the next stressful experiences in your day. List what you could do?

1>

2>

3>

What gets you out of bed in the morning? What could you begin scheduling that you could look forward to as you awake? Having positive behaviors we enjoy on a daily basis begins a foundation of happiness to offset negative experiences we have to endure.

1>

2>

3>

What are the events you have to face each day you wish you could avoid? We have tasks, people, meetings, "to do lists", projects, and expectations of others that cause us stress, bore us, or depress us. How can we start working around these obstacles to our happiness? First is being aware of the activities that stress us.

1>

2>

3>

What might be a "keystone habit" you could begin? This might be a habit that would change your life. Starting any of the 5 behaviors can affect your perspective on all your behaviors. It could be things like a positive plan to eat better, beginning an exercise routine, setting aside time to learn or be creative each day, start writing a book, enrolling in a course on something you have dreamed of learning, start a project that would make a contribution, begin teaching, spending an hour at night with a child, or …

1>

2>

3>

What is a skill(s) you could learn that would impact your career? There are skills you might not have that would pave the way to a promotion. They may be outside your job description. Some might be public speaking, computer science, leadership, creative writing, art, athletics, design, memorization techniques, podcasting, video creation, time management, or

1>

2>

3>

How could you start organizing important activities into time blocks? Time blocks allow total focus. Focus leads to "flow". Flow is our ultimate learning and creativity state. You might need the support of your superiors, co-workers, mate, or children. Which activities and hours would be most beneficial?

Which activities

1>

2>

3>

Which Hours?

1>

2>

3>

What are some areas in which you procrastinate? Procrastination creates stress and drains the energy to be creative. How could you change?

Areas of procrastination

1>

2>

3>

What changes could you make?

1>

2>

3>

Our time management can interfere with long-term growth. What are the non-important activities or distractions (phone, internet surfing, Instagram) that could be consolidated into our low energy periods to make room for important career building activities? If we prioritize learning, creativity, contribution, health, and fitness, what could we minimize?

1>

2>

3>

Our addiction to speed can interfere with long-term plans for growth. We pack too much into a day and don't leave room for real game changing personal development. What skills could you learn or obligations could you assume to begin building a long-term path to career goals? Sometimes learning on a broad base can build a better pyramid. Could we enroll in classes, get coached, have a mentor, study a curriculum, begin a health program, set some long-term goals with daily engagement? If we don't focus on just what needs to be done tomorrow, but create a framework for what we want in our lives, we get a different perspective. What could you change?

1>

2>

3>

Contribution not only stimulates oxytocin, but can be a purpose and give our life meaning. Sometimes we have to build skills to have more value or we have to decide to share what we know. Contribution is often caring and feeling connection to the people and world around us. How would you like to see the world change from sharing your experience, skills, ideas, or work? What are your values you would like to share? How could you get people not as skilled as you started? What could you learn that you could teach?

1>

2>

3>

Health supports a quality lifestyle. We often sacrifice it for short term obligations. The time we don't spend now could end up being all we think about if we allow our bodies to deteriorate. Ask someone who is suffering. What could you start to do to improve your health? Better nutrition, relaxation time, reduce stress, look for spiritual pursuits, exercise daily, support personal relationships, develop empathy and gratitude.

List some things you could begin and they might become "keystone habits"

1>

2>

3>

Imagine you are writing your book, movie, or song. You want to start a business or project. You achieved your goal and now you are going to tell others about it in your own movie or narrative. How does your story evolve? Think through how it is going to go.

What are the first things you feared and the first obstacles?

1>

2>

What are the first steps you took to overcome the starting resistance?

1>

2>

What are the challenges you encountered along the way?

1>

2>

What did you do to meet the challenges?

1>

2>

How did you feel in the process?

1>

What were the fears you experienced?

1>

2>

3>

What were the things/people/events that gave you hope along the way?

1>

2>

3>

How does your story end?

1>

How do you feel at the end of your achievement?

1>

Risk taking can be a major growth activity. Adrenaline junkies are the extreme, but their adventures do become their purpose. Extreme athletes say the dangers they face are within their capabilities and they engage for the feelings. We should try to get out of our comfort zones frequently. Just pushing our boundaries activates our happiness brain chemicals and grows us. What scares you that could grow you? Blogging, public speaking, learning difficult material, sharing what you know, building relationships, starting new processes, beginning an exercise or diet program, creating more intimate relationships, learning and sharing art (painting, music, writing, dance).

List some activities that would take you out of your comfort zone, but would grow you.

1>

2>

3>

Worry and anxiety can impede our health and our growth. Worry is an alert that we have a problem. We should spend time immediately diagnosing what worries us and how we can solve the problem(s). Anxiety is usually a fear that doesn't materialize. We have to learn to neutralize the improbabilities of anxieties becoming real. Anxiety is a full body alert.

What are some things you commonly worry about
that you could itemize and then list the ways you
will solve these issues? Paying bills, making a
good impression, completing a project, meeting a
deadline, advancing in a career, getting funding for
a project.

A common worry

1>

2>

3>

List of measures to solve this problem(s)

1>

2>

3>

What are some things that cause you anxiety?
Anxiety is more of a full body experience than
worry. Anxiety can affect digestion, prevent
thinking, kill creativity, make you irrational. Losing
your job, getting reprimanded by your boss, losing
a relationship, being embarrassed in front of co-
workers, having a project fail, not being able to
pay bills. The most important first step is to
realistically assess the likelihood of the fear
actualizing. Is the anxiety about something
unimportant? Are your precautions likely to keep
the anxiety from happening (getting to the airport 2
hours early)(starting a project way in advance of

the deadline)? Is the anxiety about something that can't be resolved (an asteroid hitting the earth)(China and the U.S. creating a global depression)?

What are some things that make you anxious? How likely are they to happen? How good is your history avoiding things you were anxious about? How prepared are you for the worst that could happen? Are you already thinking of a plan if the worst should happen?

1>

2>

3>

We have more time than we think. The first resistance a coach faces with any new prospects is their concept of their available time. We think our days are packed. Yet, unless we create time for growth and health, our lives may not be what we need. Poor health and a lack of purpose have serious consequences. We also don't assess how much time is non-productive in our days. We should begin to assess what doesn't move our lives forward. Then we might need permission or support from those in our lives to substitute what is important for what is not.

List some positive habits that need to be included in your life.

1>

2>

3>

List some activities that are a waste of time. Bad
habits, TV, social media, gossip, urgent non-
important tasks, "to do lists", email. How much
time could you create by minimizing or putting
them all together in a one-hour block? Minimizing
boring tasks frees up mind space for creativity.

1>

2>

3>

What would a perfect day look like? This is really
the focus of the Course. We want as many
meaningful, purposeful activities as possible in our
days. These activities grow us, make us healthy,
and feel purposeful.

Could you list your ideal day with the most
rewarding activities from morning until night?

1>

2>

3>

4>

5>

Add more..

From a slightly different approach. What would have to happen in your days for you to look back each day and say, "Wow, that was a good day"?

List, if different from above, what activities would be included each day to make them "Wow" days. This is your life you are building.

1>

2>

3>

4>

5>

For Businesses That Would Like Ways to Deliver the "Creating Your Own Happiness" Message

This book is a great start. It is also on Kindle.

There is/will soon be an audio version

There is/will soon be a 5 video training course

Talks to groups as key notes, company meetings, or department meetings

Group discussions

Webinars

Live Trainings once a week can lead workers through the process of setting goals and achieving change

Personal Coaching

See the website 9Climb.com for rates, programs and contact information

Email to Mark@9Climb.com

Bibliography

Habits of a Happy Brain   Loretta Graziano Breuning

The Athlete's Way   Christopher Berglund

The More Daring Life   David Berry

Managing Your Mind   Gillian Butler PH.D.

The Inner Game   Timothy Gallowey

FS.Blog   Shane Parish

The Rise of Superman   Steven Kotler

The Science of Positive Thinking   Loretta Graziano Breuning

The Power of Habit   Charles Duigg

Drive: The Surprising Truth About What Motivates Us   Daniel Pink

Go Wild   John J. Ratey and Richard Manning

Best Self, Be You Only Better   Mike Bayer

The Plan   Lyn-Genet Recitas

Move IntoThe 9 Essentials for Long Life Vitality   Anat Baniel

Younger Next Year   Chris Crowley and Henry S. Lodge

Mark Kaplan

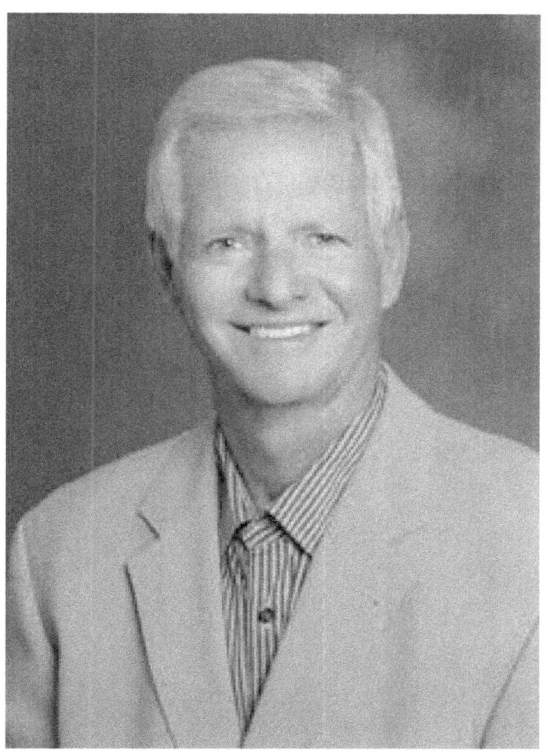

I have enjoyed years of coaching. In my real estate days, I was an office and regional manager. Coaching agents to succeed and supporting their efforts was the enjoyable part of the work. Since then, I have worked with people to improve their lives in many ways.

I enjoy interacting with people to help reach goals. I follow my own lifestyle model of continuous learning, creativity, contribution, health and exercise.

I would look forward to meeting with you and working with you on creating your optimum life.

ACE Certified Health Coach

Personal Trainer

Fitness Nutrition Specialist

Surfing Coach

Life Style Coach